VEGAN AND VEGETARIAN NUTRITION HEALTH BENEFITS

THE DANGERS OF FARM FACTORY RAISED ANIMAL CONSUMPTION
ANIMAL CRUELTY AT THE SLAUGHTERHOUSE

Mark Brohl

TABLE OF CONTENTS

INTRODUCTION

Going back in time some ten years ago, I vividly remember a week in particular that I had been questioning myself as to why I was a meat-eater. I seemed to eat it at every meal but I never really enjoyed it that much. My meat consumption would only exist in casseroles, burritos, sauces, or even a hamburger, but never a meal where there was a huge slab of beef staring at me from my plate. If I was at a high-end restaurant and they offered me the thickest, highest quality cut of "Filet Mignon" for free (this never happened) I would not take it. I would rather have a hamburger and even a Mcdonalds hamburger at that.

It was the spring of 2009 when I per-chance ran into a twenty-five-year-old friend who I had not seen in the last ten years. He was barely recognizable. I remembered him as being very out-of-shape and very overweight. He could not walk up a flight of stairs without heavy breathing and this was as of today thirty five years ago when he and I were both in our mid to late '20s. We were not the most likely of buddies at least as it came to body image. I always took pride in being in shape and still do. I don't remember why we became friends but I do know that our personalities just kind of clicked.

The guy that was standing in front of me was sleek as a cat. He looked like he could shed his sport coat and tie at any moment and break off and run a 25-mile marathon at the sound of a whistle. I remember my first words were, "Charlie, (not his real name) is that you!?" Anyway, it was great seeing him and even better seeing him in his new body and mindset. We had a great time. I asked him how he had changed so much and how he had become so healthy and vibrant. I expected to hear a long tale about serious dieting and many long strenuous work-outs with many hours in the gym and many miles logged running on a treadmill or around a track. Instead, his answer was simply, "I became a vegetarian." Ok, I thought, not really knowing what to say, but remembering my own past musings as to why I was a meat-eater.

We did not speak much more on that subject through the rest of the evening but just kind of spent time catching up. When it became time to part ways, we shook hands and promised to stay in touch. Just before leaving he handed me a napkin with 3 words on it. The words were, "Meet Your Meat". I was a bit dumbfounded but he just said, "google it" and then we parted ways.

It must have been two to three days later when I was at my computer and had a little bit of time that I decided to google "Meet Your Meat" and from then on my meat-eating days were about to come to an end. I had never seen such a haunting and graphic video. I was unable to watch it all the way through upon my first try and then only by squinting my eyes through a good portion of it. It is not a high-quality video but one with candid footage of farm-factory raised animals and actual footage of a slaughterhouse in real-time.

Farm-factories are just what they imply. They raise and roll-out animals for human consumption just like steel factories roll out steel for its purpose. The terrible conditions these animals are forced to endure throughout their miserable, prematurely shortened lives, is unbearable to witness. All of this misery will ultimately culminate in the brutal "Terror of the Slaughterhouse".

The first two chapters of this short book deal with the reality of the farm-factories that produce the meat that comes to your table and the slaughterhouse where the lives of these sentient beings come to a brutal end. The rest of the chapters deal with the health benefits of forsaking meat and adopting a healthy vegetarian diet. Some myths are shattered along the way, and America, sad to say, is truly depicted as the most prosperous country on earth yet probably the most unhealthy of any 1st world country. I love my wonderful America but am sickened as to the state of our health and how we became as such.

If you have ever suffered from health problems, or just worry that you will become the next cancer or heart attack victim, this book is for you. If you have struggled with weight gain and can't seem to ever shed the pounds and constantly go from diet to diet only to put the weight back on, this book is for you. You can shed those pounds effortlessly without diets or strenuous work-outs. If you are conscious about wrinkles and aging every time you look in the mirror, this book is for you. Wrinkles begin to disappear and the time clock turns back before your very eyes and this without conscious effort on your part - it just happens! If you want to save thousands of dollars at the grocery store and multiplied thousands of dollars because of not needing to buy astronomically priced pharmaceutical drugs, this book is for you. If you worry about the prospect of giving up your life savings for the purpose of life or death violent surgery due to a heart attack or cancer then this book is for you.

I have done extensive research over the years about these, and related topics, and have seen countless examples of the impact a mere change in the way we think about eating can have on our lives. I have over 52 published articles on related subjects and enjoy writing them and witnessing lives transformed in such a "no brainer" fashion.

In closing, I want to thank you all for taking the time to purchase and read this short book. I wish you and your loved ones and families good health, peace, long life, and happiness.

Chapter 1

THE TERROR OF THE SLAUGHTERHOUSE

" ...If slaughterhouses had glass walls, everyone would be a vegetarian." Paul and Linda McCartney

If every human being was forced to witness the heinous cruelty at the slaughterhouse and was compelled to listen to the sounds of terror emanating from these death houses, the only factory farm meat eaters left would be those who were too much an animal themselves to even be called human.

I am sure there will be those who are horrified at such a statement but that is only because they have not been made aware of the terror that permeates the very walls of a slaughterhouse or they have steadfastly closed their eyes to the truth of the incomprehensible cruelty.

If we have the slightest care or concern for our animal friends then we cannot at the same time witness the cruelties of these houses of pain and torture and continue the practice of eating "farm factory meat" without feeling a heavy burden of sadness. Therefore, if we would boast of having a reasonable amount of empathy for the wonderful animals that share our planet and yet refuse to become informed, or worse, close our eyes to these unimaginable abuses, the kindest thing that could be said about us is that we are insincere.

Let us be clear however of what it is we are refusing to become informed about and also what it is we are adamantly refusing to open our eyes and see. Of course if you already know or suspect the following explanation of atrocities in regards to the slaughter of farm factory animals and yet feel not the slightest compunction of guilt for the plight of these innocent, voiceless creatures, then certainly articles like this won't change your heart nor will the articles of far more capable writers who have gone before me. Your only hope would be to pay a visit to any slaughterhouse in America and see for yourself.

I am not going to waste your time or mine attempting to site the hour and place of each occurrence of cruelty, because if you will merely talk to a worker in a slaughterhouse, or a transporter of animals to the slaughterhouse then you will have all of the proof you need. If however, we reject the following statements without even an attempt to confirm their veracity, then surely our irresponsibility is one of the reasons that slaughterhouses in their present form still exist.

THE TRANSPORT

Many times, animals are herded from a more rural area into the city where they are loaded onto transport trucks. These poor creatures whose bodies are already spent from a life of unimaginable cruelty and horrifying living conditions are made to run to the place where they will be transported to their death. The use of red chili powder administered to the eyes is a well known method of getting them to run to their slaughter faster. There are beatings and torture all along this march to death and of course they take place in all sorts of weather conditions, from sweltering heat to bitter cold. This is the horrible road to the transport truck that will ultimately take them on their last ride.

Once placed in the truck they do not even have room to move. Fast stops and starts many times cause great injury to the animal as they are knocked around the truck and often fall on each other breaking bones and suffocating. Again, these transports often take place in extreme weather conditions and of course the animals are afforded no protection.

THE ARRIVAL

A sickening percentage of farm animals never make it to the slaughterhouse alive. The ones that do are only half alive or worse. Many already have broken limbs before they are thrown like a sack of potatoes off the truck onto the pavement. Of course this will quite often break even more bones. These animals are not in any way considered sentient beings but merely a product, such as a bale of hay, and they are treated as such. The only difference is that you don't have to kill a bale of hay.

THE SLAUGHTER

The sounds of terror that assault you and then haunt you can soften the hearts of even the cruelest of men. Terrified pigs still fully conscious, squealing and kicking are often seen being lowered into a tank of scalding water. The unimaginable is commonplace each and every hour behind slaughterhouse walls. Electric prods are used, castration, branding and docking of tails as well as de-horning which involves applying red hot irons to the calf's horns for a sustained period in order to be able to rip them out of their head. De-beaking applies scorching heat to the victim enabling their beaks to be ripped out. All of these atrocities of course are done without anesthetics. Ofttimes after stunning (although this might immobalize they are still many times conscious and can feel every bit of pain) their throats are slit and they hang their to bleed out fully aware that they are bleeding to death or they are just left to lay in their own blood and that of the slain that went before them as death slowly overtakes them. People who have worked in slaughterhouses will testify that many of these innocents are fully conscious during all of this. They are conscious and aware that they are hung by their leg upside down to bleed out and suffocate on their own blood. One worker said that "some would survive as far as the tail cutter, the belly ripper, and the hide puller. They die piece by piece." Others testify that many animals make it as far as the skinning process fully alive and conscious. They are skinned alive!

These and many more horrendous atrocities are just business as usual in the slaughterhouse.

In my estimation, the simplest solution to these horrendous practices is to quit eating farm factory meat. If you are a household of four, your decision to stop consuming intelligent animals could possibly save you around $2000.00 dollars or more per year. If you have struggled with your weight in the past, you will be pleased at how quickly pounds of fat begin to drop off when you eat a healthy vegetarian diet. Your chance of suffering a heart attack will greatly diminish as well as your chances of suffering from cancer, stroke, diabetes, and other dread diseases. Your choice to forsake eating farm factory meat will also pay great dividends in the health of our environment. Most importantly, you will be doing your part to spare a helpless animal from the terror and the cruel fate of the slaughterhouse.

MARK BROHL

Chapter 2

ANIMAL FARM FACTORIES
WHAT DOES OUR MEAT EAT?

What do you think of when you envision farm factory animals? Do you think of a fat cow in a sun-drenched pasture munching on some green grass? Or do you imagine some chickens lazing about pecking on the ground for seed outside of a beautiful red barn? These scenes look wonderful on a post card but are not the actual proceedings at farm factories.

The Reality

Animals on most farm factories are literally tormented every hour of their existence until they meet a cruel torturous fate at the slaughterhouse. These farm factories have realized that by cramming the most animals into the smallest space possible they can greatly increase their profit margins. Let me also assure you that there is absolutely no concern for the welfare of the animal when profits are in reality the only consideration. This is one of the reasons for the term "farm factory". Given this reality do you think that these animals are being fed high quality food, or do you think these factories attempt to cut costs here also?

The truth is that in the brutal farm factories never ending search for ways to lower costs and thereby increase profits, they have resorted to feeding these poor abused creatures that which is unbelievably unhealthy for them as well as the humans that consume their flesh.

What's for Dinner?

Have you ever heard of Mad Cow Disease? That is the consequence of feeding dead cows to live cows. The Federal Government has intervened a bit in this connection but cattle can still be fed blood from dead cows as well as other parts from these carcasses. Pigs, turkeys, chickens, etc., can all legally be fed the dead carcasses of their own species. And of course, these animals can be fed the carcasses of cattle, and when they die, they in turn can be fed to cows, so as you can see the cause of Mad Cow Disease has not really been stopped, but it is just a bit longer cycle now. The steak you had for dinner last night can legally be fed dead horse, dead dogs, cats, feathers, hair, hooves, blood, internal organs, and other disgusting matter.

Of course all of this (feed?) contains large traces of cow, pig, and poultry manure, as well as the drugs they have been fed such as antibiotics, (to keep these poor creatures alive under terribly crowded, unsanitary, and stress filled conditions) arsenic and hormones (to promote faster growth) and anything else that might sneak into the food they are subjected to. Many of the drugs they have been fed passes straight through their bodies without change so that you and I can ingest them with our dinner. Isn't this wonderful?

And please don't forget that our vision of Elsie the cow grazing in a lovely pasture eating what they are meant to eat (grass) is not what is happening. Besides the antibiotic and hormone rich dead animal carcasses they are fed (which they can't digest) they are also fed huge amounts of grain (which they also cannot digest) in order to fatten them up quicker for the slaughter so we can have our share of these delicacies at our next barbecue.

If you have ever wondered why the antibiotics that used to help clear up your ear infection are no longer as effective, please understand that the above practices make bacteria highly resistant to antibiotics and this is just one of the many unhealthy results of the inhumane raising of animals in farm factories.

An Informed Choice

If we choose to turn a deaf ear to these practices and continue to eat our farm factory meat because it tastes good, then there is not much anyone could say. I must admit however; it is very difficult for me to conceive of a choice for the above by any rational human being. It is even more incomprehensible when there is a simpler, far healthier, and more sterile alternative. A plant based diet is exactly what the doctor ordered. If you desire to greatly decrease your chances for heart disease, cancer, diabetes, stroke, obesity, etc., please consider the benefits of vegetarianism. But even if your own health and welfare is of no great concern to you, then at least do it for the benefit of these tortured animals that should in reality be our friends. And while you are at it, you will be simultaneously making a huge contribution to the betterment of the environment of the planet we call home. I hope we will all become informed about the reality of these farm factories and the meat we eat.

MARK BROHL

Chapter 3

VITAMIN D FROM SUNSHINE
THE SUN IS NOT YOUR ENEMY, YOUR DIET IS

The Sunscreen Industry Says The Sun Is Your Enemy -- Actually Your Enemy Is The Toxins In Your Body

Sunlight on your bare skin is the only natural way to produce vitamin D. I know these amounts to heresy when you consider the claims of the sunscreen industry, but be that as it may, God's sun is what sustains all life on this planet. Your need for the life giving rays of the sun are stronger than horseradish, but the negative hype generated by the billion dollar suncreen industry might very well have you believing that this source of life and healing is actually your enemy.

We must first understand that the diseases that, we, or our loved ones are experiencing are not coming from external sources such as the sun. Our infirmities are caused by internal issues such as a lack of antioxidants, enzymes, vitamins, minerals, fiber and whole, raw, living foods. Every natural element as well as every pharmaceutical drug is our enemy when we have starved our body and our immune system of these sources of life, but this is not a problem which God's sun has engendered, nor are any other of His natural fruits, vegetables, herbs or grains responsible for our disease. The natural world that God has created is abundant with these healing foods and by eliminating processed and refined aborations that actually claim to be foods we will protect our bodies from a world of diseases.

Vitamin D Is Free, but our Body Is A Toxic Wasteland.

Although Vitamin D might be the most important vitamin for overall health that we will ever consume, we will never need a prescription for it because it is always made available in abundance by the very rays of the sun. This fact will not change just because the multi-billion dollar sunscreen industry spends vast sums of money to make sure that we are paranoid about the sun's wonderful health giving qualities.

Our problem with the sun does not come from the sun itself but from the toxic wasteland that is our body. When the sun comes in contact with skin that is full of antioxidants and proper nutrition, it does not burn but instead produces incalculable health benefits. However, when the sun comes in contact with the average American's skin it becomes poison. This is not because the sun is poison but because we have been ingesting too much alcohol, processed food (garbage), fast food (the worst garbage), and have kept far away from fresh fruits, vegetables, nuts and seeds.

If we have ever wondered why our health and life is lived on a sub-par level and we have never considered our diet as the primary culprit, I am here to tell you that this is the reason. If we continue to deny that our diet is the main problem with our health then get ready to give away a large portion of your lifesavings to pharmaceutical companies whose drugs will never provide healing for your body, and then start saving again so you can give the rest of your lifesavings for your by-pass surgery or the dreaded immune system destroying chemotherapy.

If we do desire to experience freedom from every disorder, we have been ingloriously forced to endure then please understand that the next statin drug is not our way out of this dreadful fate. We can change our life by changing our diet. Stop eating the flesh of innocent animals (or at least farm factory animals) and stop eating as much food that comes from a fast food restaurant. Start eating fresh fruits and vegetables, whole grains, nuts and seeds that come from the soil of the earth and we will begin to see incredible changes in our health, life and attitude.

We have the power to take control over our own health and it will not be necessary to give our life savings to a physician to do so. We can start to experience perfect health through perfect nutrition. Shun all farm factory animal products and opt for organic fruits, vegetables, beans, nuts and seeds and see if one month does not change the course of your health for a lifetime. As an aside, I incorporate the term "farm factory animals" because of what they are fed, to include antibiotics, hormones, and a diet they cannot digest in order to fatten them up quickly for slaughter. They are also fed dead carcasses often times of the same species. If you love your meat at least make sure it is free range grass fed beef and although more expensive, you would save it down the line in terms of very expensive health issues.

If we refuse this natural prescription for our health and instead continue on the same path that has lead to our obesity, high blood pressure, high cholesterol, and our overall terrible health, then in the end we deserve to die a horrible death at an unreasonably young age. In the final analysis it is up to us to choose life or death.

MARK BROHL

Chapter 4

OMEGA-3 FATTY ACIDS CAN A VEGETARIAN/VEGAN GET ADEQUATE AMOUNTS?

The benefits of omega-3 fatty acids cannot be denied. It is certain that those who incorporate these essential fatty acids into their diet are aiding in their own heart protection as well as lowering the risk of heart attack, reducing their risk of stroke, and even helping to keep body weight in check. In addition, healthy omega 3 fatty acid slows the buildup of atherosclerotic plaques (hardening of the arteries) and lowers blood pressure. Besides these benefits, adequate amounts of omega-3s are also linked to brain health, joint health, support of muscle building, memory, and learning support, reduction of inflammation, anti-aging, balance of blood sugar, healthy immune system, skin health, and much more. Clearly the intake of adequate amounts of healthy omega-3 fat is critical to maintaining good health, but can vegans get adequate amounts of this essential fat? The simple answer to this question is a resounding "yes."

Of course, most of us know that some of the best sources of these essential fatty acids are fatty fish such as salmon, mackerel, tuna, and sardines. But for those of us who do not consume animal flesh there are still many sources of these vital fatty acids. Actually, the consumption of vegetarian omega-3s might be more beneficial since there are absolutely no negatives associated with their consumption. In the case of fatty fish for instance, one must also admit a high cholesterol intake as well as dangerous levels of mercury.

When it comes to a healthy plant based intake of omega-3 fatty acids these negatives are not present. Nevertheless, it is essential that vegetarians and vegans are conscious of the necessity of incorporating these wonderfully healthy omega 3 fatty acids into their diets since these fats are not produced by the human body.

In the vegetable kingdom, flaxseed is doubtless one of the finest sources of omega-3. Just one rounded tablespoon of milled flaxseed provides 2000 mg of the omega-3 alpha-linolenic acid (ALA). This is the essential fatty acid that humans cannot make. Flaxseed also provides valuable cancer fighting lignans and huge amounts of dietary fiber which cannot be said for fatty fish such as salmon, tuna, mackerel or sardines.

Other great food sources of omega-3 fatty acids include:

- -walnuts
- -Brazil nuts
- -butternuts
- -chia seeds

- -pumpkin seeds
- -flax seed oil
- -canola oil
- -hickory nuts
- -spinach
- -kale, and other green leafy vegetables
- -oat and wheat germ
- -soybean and soybean sprouts
- -tofu
- -various types of beans
- -peanuts
- -olives, and olive oil
- -spirulina
- -walnuts

The positive benefits of omega-3 fatty acids are too many to count but it is not correct to say that these essential fats are limited to those who consume animal by-products and fish. Non-animal sources of these fatty acids are numerous and therefore it is not necessary that vegetarians and vegans should be to any degree deficient in omega-3s. It is necessary, however, that those who practice a healthy vegetarian/vegan diet be conscious of their intake of these vital fats. If those of us who adhere to the healthiest diet known to man (plant based) are mindful of the need of essential omega-3 fats, we can confidently continue to shun all animal flesh while enjoying the many health benefits of a strictly plant based diet.

MARK BROHL

Chapter 5

REFINED SUGAR - A HEALTH NIGHTMARE

America has a love affair with sugar. One hundred years ago, Americans ate on average one pound of sugar per year. Today, estimates of refined sugar consumption for every American are between one quarter to one half pound per day!

Refined sugar in large quantities is found in almost every processed food we buy at the local supermarket. Sugar is added to these processed foods because it is addictive. This means that you buy more of the product because you have no choice since it is necessary to feed your addiction. High fructose corn syrup is the worst of the worst (tremendously addictive) and is found in the majority of the processed foods that we consume.

If the average American did the math, they would realize that the amount of refined sugar they are consuming is off the charts. This high sugar intake produces a continuous over-acid condition and minerals are necessarily leached from the body in order to bring the body's PH back into balance. Calcium is continually taken from the bones and teeth for the protection of the blood which has led to incredible rates of osteoporosis in this country.

Excess sugar negatively affects every organ in the human body. Sugar is initially stored in the liver and when our liver cannot process the huge amounts of sugar that we consume on a daily basis, it returns the excess to the blood stream which consequently stores the body with fatty acids that find their way to your belly, butt, breasts, and thighs.

The quality of our red blood cells are adversely affected with every ounce of sugar we ingest. Due to our abundance of refined sugar consumption the immune system is constantly weakened so that our bodies cannot respond to external attacks, and this condition has lead to unprecedented increases in diseases of all varieties including diabetes, heart disease and cancer.

Health problems associated with refined sugar consumption are numerous and include:

- -suppression of the immune system

- -disruption of the body's mineral balance

- -anxiety, depression, and difficulty in concentration

- -drowsiness

- -reduction of important high density cholesterol

- -promotion of harmful cholesterol

- -hypoglycemia

- -weakened defense against infection from bacteria

- -kidney damage

- -increased risk of heart disease

- -hinders absorption of calcium and magnesium

- -promotes tooth decay

- -promotes unhealthy stomach acids

- -speeds the aging process including wrinkles and grey hair

- -increases overall cholesterol levels

- -causes extreme weight gain

- -diabetes

- -free radicals in the bloodstream

- -liver damage

- -atherosclerosis

- -hormonal imbalance

- -hypertension

- -migraine headaches

- -formation of bacterial fermentation in the colon

These are just a few of the effects of refined sugar on the human body. Every time you buy processed food from your local supermarket you are forking over hard earned money for the privilege of making sure that your family partakes of the above listed health concerns. You should also note that the above list is very limited, and much more could be added in terms of the grave health issues caused by the consumption of refined sugar.

In this writer's opinion it is high time that we as a society evaluate our eating habits and make the necessary changes which lead to optimum health. We can significantly reduce incidences of every debilitating disease that have ravaged the American population by a new awareness and conformity to sensible dietary practices. This should begin with a major decrease in the amount of sugar we consume.

MARK BROHL

Chapter 6

ASPARTAME - IS IT SAFE OR IS IT POISON?

Aspartame is present in thousands of processed and refined foods in the supermarket that you frequent. Diet sodas, artificial sweeteners, and sugarless gum might be the most recognizable providers of this toxic substance but they are not the only sources. It is the most prevalent sweetener in more than six thousand foods, beverages, multivitamins, cereals, frozen desserts, pharmaceutical drugs, and of course artificial sweeteners.

Independently funded studies are almost unanimous in their findings that aspartame causes a host of serious health problems to include: headaches and migraines, dizziness, nausea, seizures, muscle spasms, weight gain, depression, fatigue, insomnia, blindness, loss of hearing, asthma, anxiety, vertigo, tinnitus, and more.

Chronic diseases caused by the ingestion of Aspartame include: Diabetes, fibromyalgia, lymphoma, brain tumors, multiple sclerosis, parkinson's disease, alzheimer's, epilepsy, lymphoma, and birth defects just to name a few.

Aspartame is around ten percent methanol. Methanol is wood alcohol. Wood alcohol is a deadly poison. Remember moonshine? Many skid-row alcoholics have ended up blind or dead because of this poison. Once methanol is broken down in your body, one of the by-products is formaldehyde. Formaldehyde is a deadly neurotoxin. You can of diet coke provides about 180 mg of the deadly methanol. Methanol has a very low rate of excretion once it is absorbed so it is a poison that accumulates in the body. This accumulation is almost sure to cause severe negative health effects although they might fail to be attributed to the ingestion of the methanol present in aspartame. Nevertheless, you can bet your bottom dollar that that is exactly what has caused the problems along with other bad dietary and lifestyle habits.

The health hazards of aspartame are many. If you begin to research this poison you will find an enormous list of very dangerous side effects. Actually about 75% of all the adverse reactions to food additives which are reported to the FDA are related to aspartame and some of these adverse reactions include seizures and death. You should not take my word for this but you definitely should conduct your own research into this dangerous product.

It is clear to this writer that aspartame is poison and is not safe for human consumption. It makes a lot of folks a whole bunch of money so you will have to dig just a little bit for the truth since the mainstream media will not be of any help here. They have long been owned or supported by big corporations responsible for the production, sale, and distribution of this and other very harmful chemical toxins found in our food supply. It will not, however, be difficult to ascertain the truth about this poison because aspartame has absolutely zero benefits and a boatload of bad health problems associated with it's use.

Chapter 7

WHY AMERICA LOVES PROCESSED FOOD AND HATES RAW VEGETABLES WE NEED TO RE-PROGRAM OUR TASTE BUDS

Most of us have vivid memories of our mother's admonishing us to eat our vegetables, and according to my recollection, I hated them. Actually, in retrospect I don't believe I hated vegetables, but I did hate the concoction that posed as vegetables which ended up on my plate. Certainly, they weren't lovely, fresh, organic vegetables with all of their textures and colors intact. What ended up on my plate were taken out of a plastic bag of frozen vegetables, boiled until they were rather slimy and then slathered with margarine and salt in order to make them a bit more palatable. I say this because these were some of the ingrained memories I had to deal with when I decided to become a vegetarian. My ultimate decision was based on many factors including overall health, environmental concerns, and compassion for the animals that share our planet. Nevertheless, the choice to become a vegetarian was a bit daunting due to my memories of my dislike for vegetables.

In American society today, I would venture to guess that there are a vast amount of people (maybe the majority) who have an aversion to vegetables. We are a fast-food society and as such the thought of becoming a vegetarian or vegan might be a bit scary for most. Now add to this the thought of eating most of your vegetables raw, and it is easy to see how most folks would eliminate themselves from even considering such a lifestyle.

The recommended daily amount of fresh fruits and vegetables is somewhere between five and nine servings. Since you really can't eat too many fresh fruits and vegetables, I believe nine servings or more should be the norm but that is my opinion. Most Americans, however, do not even get close to the low number, unless of course french fries and ketchup are to be considered vegetables. Or as my brother once jokingly said to me, "Chicken is the only vegetable I eat." Unfortunately, that statement was probably close to the truth for him, and I would not be surprised if that could be said for a very large number of Americans.

Many people who have studied the science of raw nutrition and have adopted it as a lifestyle didn't come to such a decision singing and dancing. Many were forced to adhere to this way of life due to health problems ranging from being morbidly obese to being told they are sick enough to die. Some of these have found the transition to raw food a major challenge, and they have struggled with issues such as the idea of raw vegetables making them want to gag, much less ever having a glimmer of hope that they might actually taste good. My own aversion to vegetables was not nearly that strong, and I did not begin to gradually adopt such a lifestyle due to immediate health concerns since I was actually in very good health, but nevertheless I had some mental hurdles to overcome upon deciding to practice a vegetarian way of life. I can also say that I am not yet 75 to 100 percent raw which is pretty much the standard for considering oneself a raw foodist. I am 100 percent vegetarian, however, and I would say that nearly 50 percent of the food I eat is raw.

Fresh Fruits and Vegetables Are Good for You -- The Standard American Diet (SAD) Is Not

If fresh fruits and vegetables were not extremely good for you it wouldn't be a problem to just leave them out of the shopping cart and stick to processed and refined foods at the grocery store and fast food hamburger joints for the other percentage of your dietary needs. As I look around, I notice that this is exactly what many Americans actually do however, hence our outbreak of obesity, diabetes, and soaring rates of cancer and heart disease.

We are a society which has become addicted to processed and refined foods, and as a society we find it almost impossible to pass up at least one visit per day to the "Golden Arches" or some other poison dispensary. Many of us begin our day with the breakfast menu at our favorite fast food joint, and then go back for lunch. At night we sit down to a T.V. dinner, a pot pie, or a take out pizza, and we wonder why we are fat and sick. We complain that our doctor bills are far too high and therefore the endless debates and fighting about how best to solve the crisis of health care in this country.

Big food business has spent a ton of money to research exactly what it is that will get you addicted to their food, and they have done a great job too. We are now addicted to sweeteners, artificial preservatives, genetically modified foods (which are really not food at all) and sugar. No wonder the thought of eating fresh fruits and vegetables makes us want to throw up. Our taste buds have been altered and we truly are a junk food addicts. I could just as easily use the term NON FOOD ADDICT because the food that we are eating out of the box, or can, or from our local fast food joint is really not food at all. It is made in a lab, and has been genetically altered.

Sugar is one of the main reasons big food business has enjoyed our supreme loyalty and all the money that goes with it. There is some variety of sweetener in literally everything that is prepared commercially. If you can't pronounce it, it is very likely some form of sweetener. The most dastardly sweetener of all is high fructose corn syrup. This might not sound that bad but please note that the word corn is not the same kind of corn you see when you go to your local grocers. This corn is genetically engineered and is used for such things as fuel as well as sweetener, but it is not edible for human consumption any longer. Of course, it is much sweeter than regular sugar and that is why if this or some other sweetener was not present in virtually every bit of food we eat, we wouldn't be back for seconds.

Big food business has made us addicts and they have literally re-programmed our taste buds so that even the thought of a fresh organic vegetable makes us queasy. Someone has termed the food we eat "frankenfood" and that is a good designation because it was made in a laboratory, but the amazing thing is that this genetically altered food gets us salivating and excited upon just smelling it, while the fresh, vibrantly colorful appearance, smell, and taste of whole living food from God's Garden makes us ill. Big food business is responsible for doing that to us and it is high time that we pull our overweight, undernourished body out of our easy chair and say NO to our soon coming heart attack. Say NO to an industry who puts profit above our nutrition or our health. Say NO to a degenerative disease and an early grave.

Americans need to take charge of their own health and quit selling it to big business. There should be no health care debate in this country because we are the most affluent society on earth and we can really choose to eat anything we want. Healthy healing food is readily available and for the most part is much cheaper to buy than the junk we have been gorging ourselves on. But even if the cost of healthy, fresh, organic fruits and vegetables were ten times higher than the poison we have been ingesting, I assure you all of that cost will be put back in our pocket when a third or more of our income is not spent on visits to the doctor and statin drugs which cannot now and never will be able to provide one iota of healing for our bodies.

If you are like most Americans, swept up in a "frankenfood" culture and almost allergic to healthy living foods, I implore you to begin to make a positive change to a diet that promotes health, healing and overall well-being, and turn your back on your artery clogging, digestion stopping, diabetes, cancer, and heart disease promoting non-food addiction. W.H. Auden wisely said that "Health is the state about which medicine has nothing to say." we can eat ourselves healthy, or we can eat ourselves to death, but please be clear that both of those choices are in our power to decide. Statistically speaking we are going to die of heart disease, cancer, stroke, or just live out our years with a degenerative and chronic disease that makes life almost unbearable. We will give a large portion of our life savings for surgery or drugs that will never heal us but will only prolong the agony. If this does not sound acceptable to you than please make the common sense choice to do something about it. Such a paradigm shift will not be easy but it WILL save your life. Choose life and whole living foods that heal the body and soul and may God richly bless your journey!

Chapter 8

GOING RAW - DO IT FOR YOUR HEALTH

Have you ever considered the beauty and bright vibrant colors of fresh produce? Fruits and vegetables of all varieties are wonderful and inviting to look at and it is these deep vibrant colors that let you know that the produce is full of antioxidants which are called poly-phenols. The brighter the color of your fruits and vegetables the more nutritious they are and the more they are able to aid in the prevention of degenerative diseases.

Now consider for a moment what happens to the colors of these beautiful bright fruits and vegetables after cooking. That's right, they lose their brightness and the colors fade like a bright red shirt or blouse that has been laundered too many times. More importantly than the fading colors, however, are the fading health benefits of these healing foods. It should be obvious just by the before and after pictures of fruits or vegetables subsequent to cooking that this tampering with the produce is in fact robbing the food of its natural health and beauty benefits.

America may very well be the most overweight country on the planet but surprisingly we are at the same time probably the most undernourished. Of course, I am not now considering countries whose populations are so poor that they do not have enough food to eat, nevertheless, their undernourishment is the very regrettable result of a lack of food whereas our American undernourishment comes from too much food. Our bodies are literally starving at the very same time that we are chowing down on our processed and refined delicacies. We are overfed and undernourished. A constant barrage of slick advertising inviting us to eat a variety of poisons makes it a necessity to start a process of deprogramming in order to counteract this sustained brainwashing that has led us to become the most unhealthy nation on earth.

Our problem is not a lack of eating but rather a lack of digesting and assimilating the vitamins and minerals in our food. This digesting and assimilating is accomplished by enzymes. Enzymes are the difference between life and death. A corpse might very well have an abundance of every essential vitamin, but what it doesn't have are life giving enzymes and therefore the vitamins are of no value. Every operation and chemical reaction of the body is accomplished through enzymes.

Metabolic enzymes make our bodies function, and digestive enzymes do just what their name implies, they aid in the digestive process of our food. Only raw, living foods are enzyme rich and therefore they not only aid in the digestive process but also provide perfect assimilation of the vitamins and minerals.

The magic number for the killing of enzymes through the process of cooking seems to be 118 degrees Fahrenheit. When food is cooked the enzymes are destroyed and your body is forced to use up it's own store of enzymes to digest and then assimilate food. This is a waste of enzymes as well as energy.

There is life in all plants, and in terms of enzymes, they are still alive when for instance an apple is plucked from a tree. The only thing that has been cut off from that apple is it's source of nutrition, but enzymatically it is very much alive. Seeds, nuts, fruits and vegetables will sprout when buried in the ground. This is proof that they are living foods. It should be mere common sense that living foods are the best choice one can ingest for the health of the body. This concept, however, is strangely unknown in our fast food, fast paced culture.

It is possible for chemist's to isolate and synthesise nutrients and vitamins found in nature but they cannot, nor will they ever be able to breathe life into them. Enzymes are responsible for this and therefore are miracles of nature, or better yet of God who created all things.

Enzymes will not survive heat, microwaving, or pasteurization. Every time food is cooked it alters the food in such a way as to destroy it's life giving properties. The only species on the planet that cook what they eat are humans. Moreover, we apply heat to almost everything we consume. We also die of some or other chronic illness before we have lived even half of our life potential and many of those years are lived in SAD health which by the way are the very initials of the STANDARD AMERICAN DIET.

Is it wise to tout the abilities of a chef who abuses food through cooking and literally alters all of the natural food's life giving qualities? Those touted as great chefs in America are those who fall into the category of food preparers who believe that raw fruits and vegetables are not inviting to the eye or the palate. The less the prepared food actually looks or tastes like the original natural produce the more the chef is touted as a master. This is very backwards thinking and contributes to the health woes of a nation who can no longer afford health care. A true master chef should be able to create recipes of living and healthful foods that have lost none of their life giving properties. A chef who has learned to create mouthwatering recipes that heal the body instead of killing it should be the only ones affirmed as masters.

When food is cooked, nutrients which keep us living and healthy are destroyed in the process. People who are conscious of their health instinctively know that processed and refined foods are lacking in healthy nutrients and so they do their best to avoid them. But why has it escaped their notice that cooked food is also processed food (the worst kind of processing) and should also be avoided as much as possible? Eating cooked food is always the equivalent of eating dead food. We hear health fanatics everywhere claiming the benefits of unprocessed food but why should food ever be processed at all?

Almost nothing in God's Garden will ever need processing before consumption. Of course, if you kill and then eat the flesh of a living being it will of course need processing (cooking and seasoning) but this ought to tell you something about the choice to eat the flesh of a dead animal. If dead animals are the main entree in the majority of the meals you consume, I can assure you that you will become a national health statistic, and not in a good way either. You will suffer chronic illness until your premature death, and you will help to bankrupt a society whose health care bill is becoming astronimical.

Eating healthy and living foods should be a no-brainer. W.H. Auden wisely said that "Health is the state about which medicine has nothing to say." A healthy life will not be gained through paying your life savings to a physician or surgeon who administers, chops, or cuts when you are knocking on death's door. A healthy life is gained and maintained by the living foods you choose to consume. Eating living foods enables your God given immune system to heal each and every disease you can conceive of.

If it is your desire to live a long and full life free of the common health concerns experienced by virtually all Americans, then I implore you to consider your diet as the culprit of your bad health and also as the means to the promotion of health, vitality, weight-loss and anti-aging. Your food is your only true source of medicine and you need to believe and then act on this fact by making healthy dietary choices. God Bless you as you learn to live in harmony with His creation.

Chapter 9

KALE - THE KING KONG OF GREENS

Kale is just about the healthiest leafy green vegetable you will ever eat and is readily available most of the year although it is actually sweeter when grown in temperatures cold enough to produce a light frost. Seasonally it is best from mid-winter through the beginning of spring. It has an earthy flavor along with a high nutritional value which is nearly unsurpassed by just about any food. It does all of this with a very minimal amount of calories.

Besides lowering cholesterol with every bite, kale is one of the best cancer fighters around and actually has extremely potent detox properties at a genetic level. There have been over 45 different flavanoids identified in this "super food" which provide a one-two punch of antioxidant and anti-inflammatory benefits. In short, kale is head and shoulders above just about any other known food in the areas of anti-oxidant, anti-inflammatory, and anti-cancer nutrients.

Kale belongs to the Brassica family, which consists of a group of vegetables such as cabbage, collard greens, Brussels sprouts and broccoli. This is a list of heavy hitters and kale is arguably the heavy weight champ of them all. It is one of the best single sources of vitamin K, and A. It is also a great source of Vitamin C, manganese, dietary fiber, copper, vitamin B6, potassium, iron, Vitamin E, Omega 3 fatty acids, phosphorous, and also one of the best sources of absorbable calcium anywhere.

It provides around 15 grams of fiber for under 200 calories. This is significantly more fiber than the average American adult consumes in a 2000 calorie day. Fiber is as essential to our bodies as it is conspicuously absent in our predominantly animal based diet which is absolutely void of fiber.

You simply cannot experience even reasonably good health if you do not up the ante on your fiber consumption and this tasty green is about the most healthy way to get your necessary daily requirement. Likewise, in terms of cholesterol fighting ability, kale is second only to collards in providing this lifesaving benefit.

With all the fuss about Omega-3 fats (and rightly so) don't forget about kale. As if all the other benefits weren't enough (and we have only scratched the surface) kale is also an excellent source of alpha-linolenic acid (ALA) which is the basic building block for all omega-3 fats. A mere 200 calories worth of this wonderful green vegetable can provide more than sixty percent of your necessary ALA requirements.

Another wonderful benefit of this wonderful vegetable is it's production of sulforaphane which is a very powerful cancer fighter that actually signals the liver to produce these cancer fighting enzymes. You will greatly lower your risk of colon cancer, lung cancer, prostate, and breast cancer, (just to name a few) if you will make this green an important part of your diet.

This King Kong of vegetables protects against and even reverses signs of aging caused by the sun, as well as protecting the eyes from damage caused by ultraviolet light. It even helps prevent cataracts and macular degeneration, when incorporated into the diet. I have seen for myself it's ability to reverse signs of aging as both my beautiful wife and I have watched wrinkles disappear, and this miraculous age reversal has occurred quite rapidly. We both try and drink about a quart of a blended "Green Smoothie" each day. These smoothies usually consist of kale (or some other green) and whatever fruit we have lying around. Fruit makes the smoothie more than palatable and even quite tasty so consuming this anti-aging superfood is really a very pleasant experience.

I truly believe that if you had a million dollars to spend in a pharmacy and/or a beauty salon you would not be able to match the health and beauty benefits of one bunch of organic kale which you should be able to purchase for around one dollar.

This wonderful food provided by nature is a one in a million vegetable and it will certainly be a major contributor to a long healthy life. Kale is unquestionably the KING KONG OF GREENS.